Copyright ©

H. QUINONES MD

All rights reserved. No part of this publication may be reproduced, distributed, or transmitted in any form or by any means, including photocopying, recording, or other electronic or mechanical methods, without the prior written permission of the publisher, except in the case of brief quotations embodied in critical reviews and certain other noncommercial uses permitted by copyright law.

Contents

Introduction 4
Osteoporosis 7
    Fast facts on osteoporosis 8
    Signs and symptoms 8
    Causes and risk factors 9
    Diet and lifestyle choices 10
    Drugs and health conditions 10
    Causes 12
    Risk factors 13
    Dietary factors 15
    Lifestyle choices 16
    Complications 17
    Prevention 18
    Tests and diagnosis 21
    DEXA test results 22
    Senile osteoporosis 23
    Bone density test for diagnosis 23
    Osteoporosis treatment 24
    Osteoporosis medications 25
    Osteoporosis natural treatments 26
    Osteoporosis diet 27
    Exercises for osteoporosis 28

Resistance exercise machines 28
Osteopenia vs osteoporosis 29
What Is Secondary Osteoporosis.. 30
CBD For Osteoporosis & Bone Health 33
Cannabidiol Used To Improve Bone health 33
Could CBD Help Patients with Osteoporosis 34
Why Can CBD Work For Treating Osteoporosis 36
What Are The Benefits Of Using CBD To Treat Osteoporosis 37
The Endocannabinoid System & Osteoporosis 38
How Can I Use CBD To Treat Osteoporosis 39
What Are Studies Saying About Using CBD For Osteoporosis 40
The Effects & Benefits of CBD 41
How Can CBD Help with Osteoporosis 41
Making Some Adjustments... 43
Science backs CBD 44
CANNABINOIDS CAN MANAGE PAIN FROM BONE DISEASES 44
ONE COUNTER EFFECT 47
Research into the suitability of CBD for osteoporosis........... 47
Final Thoughts on CBD and Osteoporosis 49

Introduction

Osteoporosis causes bones to become weak and brittle so brittle that a fall or even mild stresses such as bending over or coughing can cause a fracture. Osteoporosis-related fractures most commonly occur in the hip, wrist or spine. Bone is living tissue that is constantly being broken down and replaced. Osteoporosis occurs when the creation of new bone doesn't keep up with the removal of old bone. Osteoporosis affects men and women of all races. But white and Asian women especially older women who are past menopause are at highest risk. Medications, healthy diet and weight-bearing exercise can help prevent bone loss or strengthen already weak bones. Osteoporosis is a disease in which bones deteriorate or become brittle and fragile due to low bone mass and bone tissue loss. The condition is often referred to as a "silent disease" because you cannot feel your bones getting weaker, and many people don't even know they have the condition until after they break a bone. Osteoporosis increases the risk of fractures, particularly of the hips, spine, and wrists. In fact, osteoporosis causes an estimated 9 million fractures each year worldwide. It can lead people to become cautious and worried about everyday life, in effect wrapping themselves in cotton wool to avoid any bone fractures. Scientific research has found that cannabidiol (CBD) products may well be a good alternative form of treatment for osteoporosis. CBD works upon the body's natural endocannabinoid system, which studies have found is actually involved in bone density regulation. Osteoporosis affects around 54 million Americans. Of those 54 million, studies suggest that about one in two women, and one in four men over the age of 50 will fracture a bone because of the condition. The reason this condition is such a concern for the elderly is that most people do not know they have the condition until after they have already experienced breaking a bone because of it. Normally, our body is constantly absorbing and replaces bone tissues but the bodies of people with osteoporosis cannot replace these tissues as fast as the body is removing them. This causes porous or brittle bones. Unfortunately, there is no cure for osteoporosis, but rather there are treatments to help manage the condition and reduce the risk for fractures. This article takes a deeper look at osteoporosis, what the condition is, the traditionally used treatments, and then compares CBD with these. If you are wondering if CBD oil could be a suitable treatment for osteoporosis, then please read on for all the information you need. As the most common type of bone disease, osteoporosis affects approximately 10 million Americans, and another 44 million people have low bone density, which puts them at risk for the disease. While osteoporosis mainly affects women, men can also develop the condition. In fact, 1 in 2 women and up to 1 in

4 four men who are over age 50 will break a bone due to osteoporosis.

Osteoporosis

"Osteoporosis" literally means "porous bones." The bones become weaker, increasing the risk of fractures, especially in the hip, spinal vertebrae, and wrist.

Bone tissue is constantly being renewed, and new bone replaces old, damaged bone. In this way, the body maintains bone density and the integrity of its crystals and structure.

Bone density peaks when a person is in their late 20s. After the age of around 35 years, bone starts to become weaker. As we age, bone breaks down faster than it builds. If this happens excessively, osteoporosis results.

Osteoporosis happens when bone density decreases and the body stops producing as much bone as it did before.

It can affect both males and females, but it is most likely to occur in women after menopause, because of the sudden decrease in estrogen, the hormone that normally protects against osteoporosis.

As the bones become weaker, there is a higher risk of a fracture during a fall or even a fairly minor knock. Osteoporosis currently affects over 53 million people in the United States (U.S.).

Fast facts on osteoporosis

Osteoporosis affects the structure and strength of bones and makes fractures more likely, especially in the spine, hip, and wrists. It is most common among females after menopause, but smoking and poor diet increase the risk. There are often no clear outward symptoms, but weakening of the spine may lead to a stoop, and there may be bone pain.

A special x-ray-based scan, known as DEXA, is used for diagnosis.

Treatments include drugs to prevent or slow bone loss, exercise, and dietary adjustments, including extra calcium, magnesium and vitamin D.

Signs and symptoms

- Osteoporosis change in posture
- As the spine weakens, osteoporosis can lead to a change in posture.
- Bone loss that leads to osteoporosis develops slowly. There are often no symptoms or outward signs, and a person may not know they have it until they experience a fracture after a minor incident, such as a fall, or even a cough or sneeze.
- Commonly affected areas are the hip, a wrist, or spinal vertebrae.

- Breaks in the spine can lead to changes in posture, a stoop, and curvature of the spine.

Causes and risk factors

A number of risk factors for osteoporosis have been identified. Some are modifiable, but others cannot be avoided.

Unavoidable factors

Non-modifiable risk factors include:

- Age: Risk increases after the mid-30s, and especially after menopause.
- Reduced sex hormones: Lower estrogen levels appear to make it harder for bone to reproduce.
- Ethnicity: White people and Asians are more susceptible than other ethnic groups.
- Bone structure: Being tall (over 5 feet 7 inches) or slim (weighing under 125 pounds) increases the risk.
- Genetic factors: Having a close family member with a diagnosis of hip fracture or osteoporosis makes osteoporosis more likely.
- Fracture history: Someone who has previously experienced a fracture during a low-level injury,

especially after the age of 50 years, is more likely to receive a diagnosis.

Diet and lifestyle choices

Modifiable risk factors include:

- Eating disorders, such as anorexia or bulimia nervosa, or orthorexia
- tobacco smoking
- excessive alcohol intake
- low levels or intake of calcium, magnesium, and vitamin D, due to dietary factors, malabsorption problems, or the use of some medications
- inactivity or immobility
- Weight-bearing exercise helps prevent osteoporosis. It places stress on the bones, and this encourages bone growth.

Drugs and health conditions

Some diseases or medications cause changes in hormone levels, and some drugs reduce bone mass.

Diseases that affect hormone levels include hyperthyroidism, hyperparathyroidism, and Cushing's disease.

Research published in 2015 suggests that transgender women who receive hormone treatment (HT) may be at higher risk of osteoporosis. However, using anti-androgens for a year before starting HT may reduce this risk. Transgender men do not appear to have a high risk of osteoporosis. More research is needed to confirm this.

Conditions that increase the risk include:

- cancer
- COPD
- chronic kidney disease
- some autoimmune diseases, such as rheumatoid arthritis and ankylosing spondylitis

Medications that raise the risk include:

- glucocorticoids and corticosteroids, including prednisone and prednisolone
- thyroid hormone
- anticoagulants and blood-thinners, including heparin and warfarin
- protein-pump inhibitors (PPIs) and other antacids that adversely affect mineral status
- some antidepressant medications

- some vitamin A (retinoid) medications
- thiazide diuretics
- thiazolidinediones, used to treat type 2 diabetes, as these decrease bone formation
- some immunosuppressant agents, such as cyclosporine, which increase both bone resorption and formation
- aromatase inhibitors and other treatments that deplete sex hormones, such as anastrozole, or Arimidex
- some chemotherapeutic agents, including letrozole (Femara), used to treat breast cancer, and leuprorelin (Lupron) for prostate cancer and other conditions

Causes

Comparing the interior of a healthy bone with one that has become porous from osteoporosis

- Osteoporosis weakens bone

Your bones are in a constant state of renewal — new bone is made and old bone is broken down. When you're young, your body makes new bone faster than it breaks down old bone and your bone mass increases. Most people reach their peak bone mass by their early 20s. As people age, bone mass is lost faster than it's created.

How likely you are to develop osteoporosis depends partly on how much bone mass you attained in your youth. The higher your peak bone mass, the more bone you have "in the bank" and the less likely you are to develop osteoporosis as you age.

Risk factors

A number of factors can increase the likelihood that you'll develop osteoporosis including your age, race, lifestyle choices, and medical conditions and treatments.

Unchangeable risks

Some risk factors for osteoporosis are out of your control, including:

- Your sex. Women are much more likely to develop osteoporosis than are men.
- Age. The older you get, the greater your risk of osteoporosis.
- Race. You're at greatest risk of osteoporosis if you're white or of Asian descent.

- Family history. Having a parent or sibling with osteoporosis puts you at greater risk, especially if your mother or father experienced a hip fracture.
- Body frame size. Men and women who have small body frames tend to have a higher risk because they may have less bone mass to draw from as they age.

Hormone levels

Osteoporosis is more common in people who have too much or too little of certain hormones in their bodies. Examples include:

- Sex hormones. Lowered sex hormone levels tend to weaken bone. The reduction of estrogen levels in women at menopause is one of the strongest risk factors for developing osteoporosis. Men experience a gradual reduction in testosterone levels as they age. Treatments for prostate cancer that reduce testosterone levels in men and treatments for breast cancer that reduce estrogen levels in women are likely to accelerate bone loss.
- Thyroid problems. Too much thyroid hormone can cause bone loss. This can occur if your thyroid is overactive or if you take too much thyroid hormone medication to treat an underactive thyroid.

- Other glands. Osteoporosis has also been associated with overactive parathyroid and adrenal glands.

Dietary factors

Osteoporosis is more likely to occur in people who have:

- Low calcium intake. A lifelong lack of calcium plays a role in the development of osteoporosis. Low calcium intake contributes to diminished bone density, early bone loss and an increased risk of fractures.
- Eating disorders. Severely restricting food intake and being underweight weakens bone in both men and women.
- Gastrointestinal surgery. Surgery to reduce the size of your stomach or to remove part of the intestine limits the amount of surface area available to absorb nutrients, including calcium.

Steroids and other medications

Long-term use of oral or injected corticosteroid medications, such as prednisone and cortisone, interferes with the bone-rebuilding process. Osteoporosis has also been associated with medications used to combat or prevent:

- Seizures
- Gastric reflux
- Cancer
- Transplant rejection
- Medical conditions

The risk of osteoporosis is higher in people who have certain medical problems, including:

- Celiac disease
- Inflammatory bowel disease
- Kidney or liver disease
- Cancer
- Lupus
- Multiple myeloma
- Rheumatoid arthritis

Lifestyle choices

Some bad habits can increase your risk of osteoporosis. Examples include:

- Sedentary lifestyle. People who spend a lot of time sitting have a higher risk of osteoporosis than do those who are more active. Any weight-bearing exercise and activities that promote balance and good posture are beneficial for your bones, but

walking, running, jumping, dancing and weightlifting seem particularly helpful.
- Excessive alcohol consumption. Regular consumption of more than two alcoholic drinks a day increases your risk of osteoporosis.
- Tobacco use. The exact role tobacco plays in osteoporosis isn't clearly understood, but it has been shown that tobacco use contributes to weak bones.

Complications

How osteoporosis can cause vertebrae to crumple and collapse.

- Compression fractures

Bone fractures, particularly in the spine or hip, are the most serious complication of osteoporosis. Hip fractures often are caused by a fall and can result in disability and even an increased risk of death within the first year after the injury.

In some cases, spinal fractures can occur even if you haven't fallen. The bones that make up your spine (vertebrae) can weaken to

the point that they may crumple, which can result in back pain, lost height and a hunched forward posture.

Prevention

Good nutrition and regular exercise are essential for keeping your bones healthy throughout your life.

- Protein

Protein is one of the building blocks of bone. And while most people get plenty of protein in their diets, some do not. Vegetarians and vegans can get enough protein in the diet if they intentionally seek suitable sources, such as soy, nuts, legumes, and dairy and eggs if allowed. Older adults may also eat less protein for various reasons. Protein supplementation is an option.

- Body weight

Being underweight increases the chance of bone loss and fractures. Excess weight is now known to increase the risk of fractures in your arm and wrist. As such, maintaining an appropriate body weight is good for bones just as it is for health in general.

- Calcium

Men and women between the ages of 18 and 50 need 1,000 milligrams of calcium a day. This daily amount increases to 1,200 milligrams when women turn 50 and men turn 70. Good sources of calcium include:

- Low-fat dairy products
- Dark green leafy vegetables
- Canned salmon or sardines with bones
- Soy products, such as tofu
- Calcium-fortified cereals and orange juice

If you find it difficult to get enough calcium from your diet, consider taking calcium supplements. However, too much calcium has been linked to kidney stones. Although yet unclear, some experts suggest that too much calcium especially in supplements can increase the risk of heart disease. The Institute of Medicine recommends that total calcium intake, from supplements and diet combined, should be no more than 2,000 milligrams daily for people older than 50.

Vitamin D

Vitamin D improves your body's ability to absorb calcium and improves bone health in other ways. People can get adequate amounts of vitamin D from sunlight, but this may not be a good source if you live in a high latitude, if you're housebound, or if you regularly use sunscreen or avoid the sun entirely because of the risk of skin cancer.

Scientists don't yet know the optimal daily dose of vitamin D for each person. A good starting point for adults is 600 to 800 international units (IU) a day, through food or supplements. For people without other sources of vitamin D and especially with limited sun exposure, a supplement may be needed. Most multivitamin products contain between 600 and 800 IU of vitamin D. Up to 4,000 IU of vitamin D a day is safe for most people.

Exercise

Exercise can help you build strong bones and slow bone loss. Exercise will benefit your bones no matter when you start, but you'll gain the most benefits if you start exercising regularly when you're young and continue to exercise throughout your life.

Combine strength training exercises with weight-bearing and balance exercises. Strength training helps strengthen muscles and bones in your arms and upper spine, and weight-bearing exercises — such as walking, jogging, running, stair climbing, skipping rope, skiing and impact-producing sports — affect mainly the bones in your legs, hips and lower spine. Balance exercises such as tai chi can reduce your risk of falling especially as you get older.

Swimming, cycling and exercising on machines such as elliptical trainers can provide a good cardiovascular workout, but they're not as helpful for improving bone health.

Tests and diagnosis

A doctor will consider the patient's family history and their risk factors. If they suspect osteoporosis, they will request a scan, to measure bone mineral density (BMD).

Bone density scanning uses a type of x-ray technology known as dual-energy X-ray absorptiometry (DEXA) and bone densitometry.

Combined with the patient's risk factors, DEXA can indicate the likelihood of fractures occurring due to osteoporosis. It can also help monitor response to treatment.

Two types of device can carry out a DEXA scan:

- A central device: A hospital-based scan measures hip and spine bone mineral density while the patient lies on a table.

- A peripheral device: A mobile machine that tests bone in the wrist, heel, or finger.

DEXA test results

The results of the test are given as a DEXA T-score or a Z-score.

The T-score compares the patient's bone mass with peak bone mass of a younger person.

- -1.0 or above is normal
- from -1.0 to -2.5 suggests mild bone loss
- -2.5 or below indicates osteoporosis
- The Z-score compares the patient's bone mass with that of other people with similar build and age.

The test is normally repeated every 2 years, as this allows for comparison between results.

Other tests

A lateral vertebral assessment (LVA) may be recommended for an older patient who is more than one inch shorter than they used to be, or who has back pain that is not related to another condition.

An ultrasound scan of the heel bone is another way to assess for osteoporosis. It can be carried out in the primary care setting. It is less common than DEXA, and the measurements cannot be compared against DEXA T-scores.

Senile osteoporosis

You may have heard of senile osteoporosis. This isn't a separate type of this disease — it's simply osteoporosis that's caused by aging. As mentioned above, age is a primary cause of osteoporosis. Unless proper prevention or treatment efforts are made, your body's increasing breakdown of bone can lead to weakened bones and osteoporosis.

According to global statistics from the International Osteoporosis Foundation, about one-tenth of women aged 60 have osteoporosis, while two-fifths of women aged 80 have the disease.

Bone density test for diagnosis

To check for osteoporosis, your doctor will review your medical history and do a physical exam. They may also run tests of your blood and urine to check for conditions that may cause bone loss. If your doctor thinks you may have osteoporosis or that you're at risk of developing it, they'll likely suggest a bone density test.

This test is called bone densitometry, or dual-energy X-ray absorptiometry (DEXA). It uses X-rays to measure the density of the bones in your wrists, hips, or spine. These are the three areas most at risk of osteoporosis.

This painless test can take from 10 to 30 minutes. Learn what to expect during a bone density test and how to prepare for it.

Osteoporosis treatment

If your testing shows that you have osteoporosis, your doctor will work with you to create a treatment plan. Your doctor will likely prescribe medications as well as lifestyle changes. These lifestyle changes can include increasing your intake of calcium and vitamin D, as well as getting appropriate exercise.

There's no cure for osteoporosis, but proper treatment can help protect and strengthen your bones. These treatments can help slow the breakdown of bone in your body, and some treatments can spur the growth of new bone. Find out more about how treatment can help support the health of your bones.

Osteoporosis medications

The most common drugs used to treat osteoporosis are called bisphosphonates. Bisphosphonates are used to prevent the loss of bone mass. They may be taken orally or by injection. They include:

- alendronate (Fosamax)
- ibandronate (Boniva)
- zoledronic acid (Reclast)

Other medications may be used to prevent bone loss or stimulate bone growth. They include:

- Testosterone: In men, testosterone therapy may help increase bone density.
- Hormone therapy: For women, estrogen used during and after menopause can help stop bone density loss. Unfortunately, estrogen therapy has also been associated with increased risk of blood clots, heart disease, and certain types of cancer.
- Raloxifene (Evista): This medication has been found to provide the benefits of estrogen without many of the risks, although there is still an increased risk of blood clots.
- Denosumab (Xgeva or Prolia): This drug is taken by injection and may prove even more promising than bisphosphonates at reducing bone loss.

- Teriparatide (Forteo): This drug is also taken by injection and stimulates bone growth.
- Calcitonin salmon (Fortical and Miacalcin) This drug is taken as a nasal spray and reduces bone reabsorption. Talk to your doctor about any increased risk of cancer with this drug.
- Prescription medication is the most aggressive way to treat osteoporosis. Learn about other medications used to treat osteoporosis, as well as possible side effects.

Osteoporosis natural treatments

Because osteoporosis medications can have side effects, you may prefer to try other treatments instead of medication.

Several supplements, such as red clover, soy, and black cohosh, may be used to help promote bone health and ease the symptoms of osteoporosis. However, before using these supplements, be sure to talk to your doctor or pharmacist. This is for two main reasons:

There are few, if any, studies supporting the use of these supplements for treating osteoporosis. As a result, we don't have proof that they work.

These supplements can cause side effects, as well as interact with medications you're taking. You'll want to make sure you know what side effects could occur, and if you're taking any medications that could interact with the supplement.

All of that said, some people report good results with natural treatments. Learn more about the natural treatment options available, as well as the risks associated with them.

Osteoporosis diet

In addition to your treatment plan, an appropriate diet can help strengthen your bones.

To keep your bones healthy, you need to include certain nutrients in your daily diet. The most important ones are calcium and vitamin D. Your body needs calcium to maintain strong bones, and it needs vitamin D to absorb calcium. Other nutrients that promote bone health include protein, magnesium, vitamin K, and zinc.

To learn more about an eating plan that's right for you, talk to your doctor. They can advise you on your diet, or refer you to a registered dietitian who can create a diet or meal plan for you. In the meantime, learn more about which nutrients you should focus on and those you should avoid, and take a look at a sample seven-day osteoporosis diet plan.

Exercises for osteoporosis

Eating right isn't the only thing you can do to support the health of your bones. Exercise is very important as well, especially weight-bearing exercises.

Weight-bearing exercises are performed with either your feet or your arms fixed to the ground or another surface. Examples include:

- climbing stairs
- resistance training, such as:
- leg presses
- squats
- pushups
- weight training, such as working with:
- resistance bands
- dumbbells

Resistance exercise machines

These exercises help because they cause your muscles to push and pull against your bones. This action tells your body to form new bone tissue, which strengthens your bones.

This isn't your only benefit from exercise, however. In addition to its many positive effects on weight and heart health, exercise can also improve your balance and coordination, which can help you avoid falls.

Always check with your doctor before starting any new exercise program. Once they give you the go-ahead, try these eight bone-strengthening exercises that you can do at home.

Osteopenia vs osteoporosis

Bone mineral density that is lower than normal but not low enough to be considered osteoporosis is called osteopenia.

Osteopenia shares the same risk factors as osteoporosis, and it raises the risk of developing osteoporosis. But not everyone who has osteopenia goes on to develop osteoporosis.

Generally, treatment for osteopenia includes weight-bearing exercise, adequate intake of calcium and vitamin D, and other lifestyle measures.

If your doctor tells you that you have osteopenia, you may think you misheard the word "osteoporosis." However, osteopenia is a separate condition from osteoporosis.

Unlike osteoporosis, osteopenia is not a disease. Rather, it's the state of having low bone density. With osteopenia, your bones aren't as dense as normal, but they're not as weakened as they are if you have osteoporosis.

The main risk factor for osteopenia is older age. Your bone density peaks at age 35, and after that, it can lessen as you get older.

In many cases, osteopenia can lead to osteoporosis, so if you have osteopenia, you should take steps to strengthen your bones. Find out more about osteopenia and ways to prevent it.

What Is Secondary Osteoporosis

Sometimes osteoporosis is caused by a medical condition or treatment that affects bone mass and causes bone loss. This is called secondary osteoporosis. Some disorders can also cause the bone marrow cavity to expand at the expense of the trabecular bone — the inner layer of bone that has a spongy, honeycomb-like structure. When this happens, the trabecular bone loses some of its strength.

Diseases and disorders that can cause secondary osteoporosis may include:

- Serious kidney failure
- Cushing's disease
- Liver impairment
- Anorexia nervosa and bulimia
- Rheumatoid arthritis
- Celiac disease
- Multiple sclerosis
- Chronic obstructive pulmonary disease
- Scurvy
- Hyperparathyroidism
- Hyperthyroidism
- Diabetes
- Hypercortisolism
- Thalassemia
- Multiple myeloma
- Leukemia
- Metastatic bone diseases

The following drugs or chemicals can also cause osteoporosis:

- Corticosteroid therapy
- Lithium
- Barbiturates
- Antacids containing aluminum

- Tobacco (when used excessively)
- Alcohol (when used excessively)

Treatment for secondary osteoporosis can be complex and may focus on treating the underlying condition or disease causing it. Other methods may include those used to prevent osteoporosis from developing.

CBD For Osteoporosis & Bone Health

Osteoporosis refers to a medical condition where human bones become brittle and fragile after losing some tissues. Naturally, bones are made of collagen, protein, and calcium. All these make bones strong and healthy. However, when a person has osteoporosis, they have very weak and fragile bones. These suffer significant effects or fractures due to a minor impact. The fractures happen due to collapsing or cracking of the bones. Osteoporosis or poor bone health is associated with problems like hip fracture and the spin vertebrae compression fracture. Hips, wrists, ribs, and spine are all areas where bone fractures can occur due to osteoporosis. Basically, osteoporosis-related fractures occur on any skeletal bone.

Cannabidiol Used To Improve Bone health

Although research is still underway, researchers hold the view that CBD can be a promising therapeutic aid for osteoporosis.

Here are some of the things that scientists have established so far:

- Cannabinoid receptors are present in the bone cells. These are CB1, CB2, and orphan receptor GPR55. Studies show that endocannabinoids and

these receptors play a role in osteoporosis development.
- Researchers suppressed the resorption of bones by blocking these receptors in adult mice. The effect was increased bone mass and protection of the mice against further bone loss. As such, they suggest the use of inverse antagonists/agonists of the receptors like CBD to combat osteoporosis.
- In another study, blocking GPR55 effect led to an increase in trabecular or spongy bone and cortical or outer surface. The mice who had their GPR55 receptors knocked out, became fatter and had better protection against bone loss that relates to age. Therefore, scientists are concluding that administering CBD can be beneficial for patients with osteoporosis.

Could CBD Help Patients with Osteoporosis

Generally, this includes a combination of supplementing diet with calcium and vitamin D, exercising (specifically weight training), and pharmaceutical osteoporosis medications, which are meant to slow down the breakdown of bones, to help maintain density. However, these treatments can come with side effects like esophageal ulcers, irregular heartbeat, calcium deficiencies, rashes, joint, bone and muscle pain, among other things.

Luckily for patients with osteoporosis, a new possible treatment – and even a potential for a cure – might have been found in cannabidiol. CBD is known best for treating epilepsy in children, but it is also effective for numerous conditions found most commonly in seniors. A handful of studies have investigated the efficacy of CBD for osteoporosis and they have found that the endocannabinoid system may play a larger part in bone health that anyone had guessed.

One study found that mice with cannabinoid receptor deficiencies have a normal peak bone mass – but that they are likely to develop age related osteoporosis. In the end, this study found that cannabinoid receptors play an important role in bone remodeling and the pathology of joint disease – which points to its potential as a treatment for osteoporosis.

Another study done on rats found that CBD may lead to improved fracture healing, based on the fact that the maximal load on the rats' bones increased significantly after treatment with CBD. Other studies, including "Cannabinoids and the Skeleton: From Marijuana to Reversal of Bone Loss" and "Endocannabinoids and the Regulation of Bone Metabolism" have found that bone loss can be prevented and even reversed by stimulating the endocannabinoid receptors within bones.

For those who are trying to find a solution to strengthen their bones, CBD may prove to be a safe addition to your treatment. It has few unwanted effects – generally dry eyes and mouth – and is completely nontoxic, making it safe for anyone to try in conjunction with their current treatments, with only the potential to benefit from the herbal extract.

Why Can CBD Work For Treating Osteoporosis

Over the past few decades, researchers have found out the presence of some cannabinoid receptors such as CB1 and CB2 in bone tissues. Indeed, these elements play an essential role in your bone health. CB2 is expressed predominantly in osteoclasts (bone-resorbing cells) and osteoblasts (bone-forming cells). This kind of cannabinoid receptor is necessary for the regulation of your bone metabolism. Physiologically, it is important to keep a balance between osteoclasts and osteoblasts as it would maintain an optimum bone health. As people age, this balance would be impaired, and result in a loss of bone density and Osteoporosis.

CB2 agonists like CBD could be used to modulate the functions of these receptors. They can improve the activity and count of osteoblasts while inhibiting the expression of osteoblasts and proliferation of osteoclasts. These elements facilitate can also stimulate the formation of Endocortical bones, suppress bone losses and maintain a normal mass of bone. CB1 receptors, on the other hand, can be activated to inhibit a chemical known as norepinephrine. This element might delay the formation of your bones, adjust the rate of reabsorption and lead to some bone issues.

Recent studies have proven that the use of CBD oils can have positive effects on these receptors, thus alleviating symptoms as well as slowing the progression of Osteoporosis.

What Are The Benefits Of Using CBD To Treat Osteoporosis

Over the years, studies have proven that CBD products have 2 distinct benefits in osteoporosis treatments. Firstly, it would negatively modulate CB2 and CB1 receptors, thus reducing their capability of binding to agonists, a compound which activates them. This is often called the entourage effect, meaning that CBD helps to reduce the effects of other compounds that serve as the same cannabinoid receptors.

What's more, CBD can inhibit several enzymes such as FAAH and increase the effects that they would exert on these cannabinoid receptors. As a result of these effects, researchers have suggested that CBD is effective and helpful in lowering the risks of osteoporosis and enhancing the health of your endocannabinoid system within the bones.

The Endocannabinoid System & Osteoporosis

The Endocannabinoid System plays an essential role in the regulation of osteoclast and osteoblast activities. This means if any problem happens in this area, it might lead to a number of conditions, including osteoporosis. There is also evidence to show your endocannabinoid system might determine the development of a low bone mass. Indeed, a lack of the endocannabinoid receptors in your brain has been linked to a higher turnover of bone. Essentially, your body might keep "retiring" old bone cells without producing enough new ones for replacement. However, if these receptors could be stimulated with the help of CBD, the bones are more likely to maintain its function even after many years. In general, the Endocannabinoid System consists of cannabinoid receptors that are activated by several elements like CBD. The endocannabinoids are basically generated and degraded by a few types of enzymes, this giving this system a role in controlling some essential activities. Consequently, reduced numbers of endocannabinoid receptors are linked to the development of osteoporosis.

How Can I Use CBD To Treat Osteoporosis

CBD oils are available in various forms and concentrations, including liquid or thick paste hemp oil, capsules, gum or candy, salves, sprays or drops, and vapor. As a rule of thumb, the dosage of CBD products for osteoporosis treatments can vary a lot as we are not the same in terms of medical conditions and level of intensity. The following of any guide is just for your reference. In general, it is advisable to start small and increase gradually until you get the desired results. It's important to remember that every person is different and everyone's reaction to CBD is different. The recommended dosage from each product can differ greatly, creating some confusion. Dosage may be different depending on the percentage of CBD oil you are using. On an average, 25mg of CBD a day is effective for most people. For strong symptoms, increase the dose slowly over a week. This, of course, is different for every patient. For more details about dosage, see our post on CBD dosage.

What Are Studies Saying About Using CBD For Osteoporosis

A recent study by French scientists has suggested that human bones come with a higher level of endocannabinoids and ligands than brain cells. Also, a naturally generated cannabinoid in our body named Anadamide could have an effect on the bone tissues. Anadamide helps to bind to those CB2 receptors. They also pointed out that CBD can imitate Anadamide, thus positively affecting bone health in those people who suffer from osteoporosis.

Another study by Idris Al focused on the important part of cannabinoid receptors in treating osteoporosis. The results suggested that CBD is likely to affect bone metabolism and ligands. Therefore, these products can be used for bone issues as it may be applied to exploit the cannabinoid receptors for targeting anabolic therapy and anti-resorptive.

A published study in 2015 by researcher Kogan Niemand has found that when mice were treated with CBD oil, the maximal loads on their bones significantly increased. Also, he discovered that CBD could speed up the process of healing fractures or broken bones.

The Effects & Benefits of CBD

Currently, the approved medications that potentially relieve and prevent osteoporosis are bisphosphonates. However, these drugs have serious or moderate side effects on the patients. Among the side effects of bisphosphonates include abnormal heart rate, nausea, esophageal inflammation, and jaw bone damage. Although some patients tolerate the side effects of these medications, they don't enjoy the therapeutic aid benefits at the end. That's because patients are likely to develop brittle bones or fractures after five or more years even after undergoing successful therapeutic aid.

Considering these serious, undesirable side effects as well as the inefficacy of the available therapeutic aids, CBD is seen as an effective and safer alternative. Some medical researchers and patients are already recommending CBD for osteoporosis. Currently, there are many CBD products that can be used to potentially relieve this condition. Take time to learn about these products on this website to make a more informed buying decision.

How Can CBD Help with Osteoporosis

Medical research has discovered that humans have cannabinoid receptors in their bone cells. The most relevant of these receptors in health terms are CB1, CB2, and GPR 55. Further research has found that cannabinoid receptors are vital for regulating bone metabolism. The CB2 receptor is expressed in osteoclasts (also known as bone reabsorbing cells) and osteoblasts (also known as bone-forming cells). The balance between the two is critical to the process of optimal bone health maintenance.

There's no denying that getting older changes our bodies, no matter how much we try to maintain our health. As people age, their bones become weaker and weaker. Bones start to lose their density, which can make them lighter and less resilient to pressure or trauma. A loss of bone mass can lead to anything from constant broken bones to structural deformities in the spine. Osteoporosis and low bone mass threaten 44 million people in the United States alone, but there may be a solution besides getting more calcium into your daily diet. CBD oil has been shown to promote bone health by stimulating new growth. Learn more the condition and about how CBD may be able to help those at risk for osteoporosis. Despite CB2's importance, studies on animals deficient in the CB1 receptor showed that they have reduced bone formation and increased bone resorption. CB2-deficient animals show age dependent low bone density along with bone loss and associated fractures. CBD is an 'agonist' of the CB1 and especially the CB2 receptors. An agonist is defined as a "substance which initiates a physiological response when combined with a receptor." In any case, CB2 agonists like CBD are capable of modulating the functions of the receptors, increase osteoblast count and inhibit osteoclast precursor proliferation. In layman's terms, CBD can help increase bone formation, reduce bone loss and aid the body in its mission to maintain normal bone mass.

Making Some Adjustments

Bone health is dependent on both the CB1 and the CB2 receptors in your cells. (THC is the ingredient in cannabis that stimulates the CB1 cells while CBD works best with your CB2 receptors.) Activation of the CB1 receptors inhibits a chemical called norepinephrine. This blockage can put your bone formation on a different schedule of formation, adjusting the reabsorption rate so you can keep the cells you already have. But the CB2 receptors that are activated appear to actually stimulate bone growth while also slowing down your reabsorption rate. Animal studies have already concluded that rats with broken bones who were treated with CBD oil healed far faster than those who weren't. By treating the bones with CBD oil, you give yourself a better fighting chance against chronic pain from osteoporosis.

Science backs CBD

A study by Kogan et al. which was published in 2015, found that when rats were treated with CBD, the maximal load on the bones increased significantly. The team also found that CBD speeds up the process of fracture healing. A study by Bib and Zimmer, which was published in 2007, also showed that CBD excels when it comes to healing broken bones. Within eight weeks, the rodents in the study experienced faster healing in their femoral bone.

As this test involved a synthetic marijuana compound, we have to be wary of the results but it is still important because it is a preclinical study. It was conducted by Zimmer, Bib, and Melamed and published in 2009. In the study, the scientists found that CBD not only stopped bone loss, it also helped to prevent it.

CANNABINOIDS CAN MANAGE PAIN FROM BONE DISEASES

Talking about bone diseases, the first threat is Arthritis, which indicates any disorder that affects joints with pain, stiffness, swelling and reduced mobility. There is no cure both for osteoarthritis, a degenerative joint disease occurring with age, and rheumatoid arthritis, which is an autoimmune disorder. Other types of rheumatic diseases also have no effective therapies. Pain is a common symptom in all types of arthritis. Prescription painkillers can lead to tolerance, harmful side effects, and addiction while trying to manage arthritis pain. Many patients die because the suppressive action on the central nervous system caused by opiates. Cannabis-based products are now used by patients as a treatment for arthritis because they can reduce pain and swelling. cannabinoid receptors osteoarthritis pain therapies cannabis CBD Scientific evidence from both lab research and human trials suggests that the whole cannabis compounds have therapeutic action in the treatment of these kinds of chronic pain. This 2014 study continues the research on the role of the endocannabinoid system in the perception of pain in osteoarthritis conditions, while this 2016 research indicates that topical CBD applications actually relief arthritis pains and inflammation without causing evident adverse effects.

We also have studies indicating that our nerves are full with cannabinoid receptors, and that peripheral CB1 receptors may be important targets in controlling osteoarthritis pain. The cannabinoid receptors are today targets for both rheumatoid arthritis and osteoarthritis pain treatments, as confirmed by this 2008 study. This 2014 study proves the involvement of the endocannabinoid system in modulating osteoarthritis pain. The CBD receptor CB2 also regulates pain responses in osteoarthritis of the knee joint, according to this 2013 research.

From lab to pharmacy, GW Pharmaceuticals, the British company specialized in cannabinoids medicines, also demonstrated on clinical trials that its cannabis-based patented compound Sativex showed a "significant analgesic effect in the treatment of pain caused by rheumatoid arthritis, and caused a significant suppression of the disease activity". GW Pharmaceuticals also holds a patent for the therapeutic use of CBG as a treatment for osteoporosis. CBG, or Cannabigerol, is not psychoactive and it is found in little quantities in cannabis plants. Its properties are currently being examined as bone-healing agents.

Science also started to consider CBD as a specific anti-arthritic substance, as this study suggest. Another recent research concludes that a CBD-derived synthetic cannabinoid might represent a potential novel drug for rheumatoid arthritis. The action of a CBD topical applications on rheumatoid arthritis is also analyzed in a 2016 research on rats indicating an evident relief in arthritis pains and inflammation.

ONE COUNTER EFFECT

We recently wrote about how cannabis can reduce pain and inflammation from arthritis. Unfortunately, we also have to mention that a recent study in the American Journal of Medicine has found that very frequent cannabis smokers are more likely to have lower body weight and broken bones. Within the participant pool of this study, 170 adults used cannabis for recreational purposes, while 114 were cigarette smokers who did not use cannabis. Heavy cannabis users showed a lower body weight and body mass index (BMI) than non-users, which might be good or bad. For sure bad is the fact that fractures seemed to be more common in heavy potheads compared to dumbass tobacco smokers. Scientists measured the bone density of the study participants, finding that heavy cannabis users had a reduction in bone mineral density. This causes a future risk of osteoporosis and fractures.

Research into the suitability of CBD for osteoporosis

The scientific research carried out into the effectiveness of CBD as an osteoporosis prescription so far has had immensely positive results. Here are the details of a few:

One study* used targeted inactivation of either the CB1 or CB2 receptors upon mice. With both groups, they found the mice had normal peak bone mass but suffered from age-related osteoporosis. These results show the cannabinoid receptors play an important role in bone remodeling.

Another study* followed up the findings that cannabinoid receptors are involved with bone mass regulation by looking at the effects of THC and CBD on rat femurs. They found CBD increased the maximal loads and work-to-failure rate of the rat femurs. THC did not have the same positive effect. From this, they concluded CBD enhances the healing of femurs and strengthens them.

In a preclinical trial, scientists created a synthetic CB2-specific agonist which affected the body in a very similar way to how CBD works. They found it rescues bone loss. From these results, they concluded that cannabinoid-based treatments should be used to combat osteoporosis.

Final Thoughts on CBD and Osteoporosis

The federally illegal status of marijuana makes accurate research difficult but we hope scientists are given access to industrial hemp at the very least. Hemp contains large amounts of CBD and no THC, the most famous high-inducing compound of weed.

It is no exaggeration to say that osteoporosis is capable of ruining your life. If you don't succumb to fractures and broken bones, the harmful pharmaceuticals you take to prevent bone mass could do as much damage as the condition itself.

Existing research on CBD already suggests that this all-natural osteoporosis treatment is superior to Big Pharma's offerings in almost every single way. The body naturally produces cannabinoids and by introducing CBD and others, you could help your body fight back against bone loss and keep osteoporosis at bay for a lot longer. If you already have the condition, CBD could prevent further bone loss and perhaps help the body create more bone.

Made in United States
Troutdale, OR
02/19/2024